Copyright © 2020 by Anna Granta

All rights reserved. This book or any portion thereof may not be reproduced or used in any manner whatsoever without the express written permission of the author except for the use of brief quotations in a book review.

First Printing, 2020
ISBN 978-1-71658-211-0

Please send any inquiries to
anna.granta@gmail.com

How to use this journal

Ideally you will fill this journal in every evening. The best way to remember is to tie it onto an existing habit. For example, fill it in right after dinner or just before you brush your teeth.

Occasionally you will forget because you are only human. Don't worry about it and don't beat yourself up. Just fill in as much as you remember, when you realise. Forgive yourself and keep going.

Decide when you will journal and write it down below:

I _________________ intend to fill out this journal each day right before/after I

____

Once a week, you will set aside a bit more time so that you can reflect on the past week and plan for the coming week.

I will reflect and plan for the week on ___________day at _______________________.

At the back of this journal is space to record your medical appointments, changes in symptoms and resources.

Week 1
A place to grow from

This week is about simplicity. You will cut out everything you don't need, to create time for healing. Practice saying 'not yet'.

What social activities will you say 'not yet' to?

____

____

____

What unhealthy food and drink will wait?

____

____

____

What work or house chores will you say 'not yet' to?

____

____

____

Goals and motivation

Life isn't all about denying yourself. Write down ten things which you can still enjoy while you are recovering.

____

____

____

____

____

____

____

____

And the three things you are most looking forward to doing again once you recover.

____

____

____

Daily record

Date: ___________

Rate your mood, from 1-5.

Describe your physical symptoms.

What did you eat and drink?

What physically, mentally or emotionally strenuous activities did you do?

How well did you sleep, from 1-5?

Daily record   Date: _________

Rate your mood, from 1-5. ☐

Describe your physical symptoms.

What did you eat and drink?

What physically, mentally or emotionally strenuous activities did you do?

How well did you sleep, from 1-5? ☐

Daily record   Date: ________

Rate your mood, from 1-5.

Describe your physical symptoms.

What did you eat and drink?

What physically, mentally or emotionally strenuous activities did you do?

How well did you sleep, from 1-5?

Daily record

Date: ___________

Rate your mood, from 1-5.

Describe your physical symptoms.

What did you eat and drink?

What physically, mentally or emotionally strenuous activities did you do?

How well did you sleep, from 1-5?

Daily record   Date: _________

Rate your mood, from 1-5.

Describe your physical symptoms.

What did you eat and drink?

What physically, mentally or emotionally strenuous activities did you do?

How well did you sleep, from 1-5?

Daily record   Date: _________

Rate your mood, from 1-5.

Describe your physical symptoms.

What did you eat and drink?

What physically, mentally or emotionally strenuous activities did you do?

How well did you sleep, from 1-5?

Daily record

Date: __________

Rate your mood, from 1-5.

Describe your physical symptoms.

What did you eat and drink?

What physically, mentally or emotionally strenuous activities did you do?

How well did you sleep, from 1-5?

Week 2
Trial and learn

Last week you noticed how your body responded to doing less. This week you will change one thing and notice what effect that has. To work out what is helping and what is not, avoid making lots of changes at once (unless your doctor recommends them). Pick one thing and do it consistently for a week.

You can use one of the ideas on the next page or come up with your own.

What one change will you try this week?

____

What result do you hope for?

____

____

____

Do you need to prepare, for example by buying equipment?

____

____

____

Menu of options

Here is a list of things you can try which may help you manage your covid symptoms. Not all suggestions will be right for you. If in any doubt about which are suitable, consult your doctor.

Experiment	Date	Result
Breathing exercises		
Meditation		
Probiotics		
Perrin Technique		
Yoga		
Diet changes		
Screen detox		
__________		
Food supplements		
__________		
__________		
Walking		
Other exercise		
__________		
__________		
Other		
__________		

Daily record   Date: _________

Rate your mood, from 1-5.

Describe your physical symptoms.

What did you eat and drink?

What physically, mentally or emotionally strenuous activities did you do?

How well did you sleep, from 1-5?

Daily record   Date: _____________

Rate your mood, from 1-5.

Describe your physical symptoms.

What did you eat and drink?

What physically, mentally or emotionally strenuous activities did you do?

How well did you sleep, from 1-5?

Daily record   Date: _________

Rate your mood, from 1-5.

Describe your physical symptoms.

What did you eat and drink?

What physically, mentally or emotionally strenuous activities did you do?

How well did you sleep, from 1-5?

Daily record

Date: _____________

Rate your mood, from 1-5.

Describe your physical symptoms.

What did you eat and drink?

What physically, mentally or emotionally strenuous activities did you do?

How well did you sleep, from 1-5?

Daily record

Date: ___________

Rate your mood, from 1-5. ☐

Describe your physical symptoms.

What did you eat and drink?

What physically, mentally or emotionally strenuous activities did you do?

How well did you sleep, from 1-5? ☐

Daily record

Date: _________

Rate your mood, from 1-5.

Describe your physical symptoms.

What did you eat and drink?

What physically, mentally or emotionally strenuous activities did you do?

How well did you sleep, from 1-5?

Daily record   Date: _________

Rate your mood, from 1-5.

Describe your physical symptoms.

What did you eat and drink?

What physically, mentally or emotionally strenuous activities did you do?

How well did you sleep, from 1-5?

Week 3
Reflect and choose

Over the last week you committed to one change. If you stuck to your commitment for the full week then congratulations! I hope your change gave you the result you hoped for. Whether or not you feel any better, you have demonstrated to yourself that you are committed to your healing. That mindset will produce change eventually.

If you were not able to keep up with your change last week, then please be kind and forgiving towards yourself. You have a choice. Do you want to try the same change again this week, or pick something different?

Did you stick to your change for a week?

____

What result did you see?

____

____

____

Do you plan to continue this change?

____

What new change will you make this week?

____

Gratitude

Being ill is hard, it's important to look after your mental health as well as your physical wellbeing. Keeping a gratitude journal is a simple yet powerful way to support your mental health.

if that isn't enough, there is evidence that gratitude practices improve happiness, physical health and sleep quality. Finally, we remember what we focus on and what we write down. This season of your life will pass and when you look back on it you will remember the good moments if you record them.

If you feel you have nothing to be grateful for, look back at your list of ten enjoyable things from week one and start doing them.

Where will you keep your gratitude journal?

____

When will you fill it out each day?

____

What three things are you grateful for today?

____

____

____

Daily record   Date: __________

Rate your mood, from 1-5.   ☐

Describe your physical symptoms.

What did you eat and drink?

What physically, mentally or emotionally strenuous activities did you do?

How well did you sleep, from 1-5?   ☐

Daily record   Date: _________

Rate your mood, from 1-5.

Describe your physical symptoms.

What did you eat and drink?

What physically, mentally or emotionally strenuous activities did you do?

How well did you sleep, from 1-5?

Daily record

Date: _____________

Rate your mood, from 1-5.

Describe your physical symptoms.

What did you eat and drink?

What physically, mentally or emotionally strenuous activities did you do?

How well did you sleep, from 1-5?

Daily record

Date: _________

Rate your mood, from 1-5.

Describe your physical symptoms.

What did you eat and drink?

What physically, mentally or emotionally strenuous activities did you do?

How well did you sleep, from 1-5?

Daily record   Date: ___________

Rate your mood, from 1-5.

Describe your physical symptoms.

What did you eat and drink?

What physically, mentally or emotionally
strenuous activities did you do?

How well did you sleep, from 1-5?

Daily record   Date: _________

Rate your mood, from 1-5.

Describe your physical symptoms.

What did you eat and drink?

What physically, mentally or emotionally strenuous activities did you do?

How well did you sleep, from 1-5?

Daily record   Date: ___________

Rate your mood, from 1-5.

Describe your physical symptoms.

What did you eat and drink?

What physically, mentally or emotionally
strenuous activities did you do?

How well did you sleep, from 1-5?

Week 4
Acceptance

"Accept what is, let go of what was, and have faith in what will be."

Worrying and hiding from your situation are understandable, but they take energy and can't change where you are in your recovery journey.

What do you find hard to accept about your illness?

____

____

____

Imagine that you did accept these things. What would you do differently?

____

____

____

What scares you about doing what you just wrote?

____

Could these changes be worth the fear?

____

Weekly reflections

Did you stick to your plan last week?

____

What was the result, will you continue?

____

Look back over your weekly gratitude
journal. What stands out?

What new change will you try this week?

____

What result do you hope for?

____

____

____

Do you need to prepare?

____

____

____

Daily record

Date: __________

Rate your mood, from 1-5.

Describe your physical symptoms.

What did you eat and drink?

What physically, mentally or emotionally strenuous activities did you do?

How well did you sleep, from 1-5?

Daily record

Date: _____________

Rate your mood, from 1-5.

Describe your physical symptoms.

What did you eat and drink?

What physically, mentally or emotionally strenuous activities did you do?

How well did you sleep, from 1-5?

Daily record

Date: _________

Rate your mood, from 1-5.

Describe your physical symptoms.

What did you eat and drink?

What physically, mentally or emotionally strenuous activities did you do?

How well did you sleep, from 1-5?

Daily record   Date: _________

Rate your mood, from 1-5.

Describe your physical symptoms.

What did you eat and drink?

What physically, mentally or emotionally strenuous activities did you do?

How well did you sleep, from 1-5?

Daily record   Date: _________

Rate your mood, from 1-5.

Describe your physical symptoms.

What did you eat and drink?

What physically, mentally or emotionally strenuous activities did you do?

How well did you sleep, from 1-5?

Daily record

Date: _________

Rate your mood, from 1-5.

Describe your physical symptoms.

What did you eat and drink?

What physically, mentally or emotionally strenuous activities did you do?

How well did you sleep, from 1-5?

Daily record   Date: _________

Rate your mood, from 1-5. ☐

Describe your physical symptoms.

What did you eat and drink?

What physically, mentally or emotionally strenuous activities did you do?

How well did you sleep, from 1-5? ☐

Week 5
Variety

Being ill for a long time can be very monotonous, even boring. Even in your illness it's possible for you to have new experiences and notice new things about yourself and the world around you. Varity is a beautiful thing and you shouldn't wait untill you are well to enjoy it.

This week, change your environment and notice the changes happening in the natural world around you.

How will you change your enviroment, for example, use a different room or put up a poster?

____

Go outside (or watch from a window or webcam). What do you see that wasn't there last week?

____

____

____

What new food will you try this week?

____

Weekly reflections

Did you stick to your plan last week?

____

What was the result, will you continue?

____

Look back over your weekly gratitude
journal. What stands out?

What new change will you try this week?

____

What result do you hope for?

____

____

____

Do you need to prepare?

____

____

____

Daily record   Date: _________

Rate your mood, from 1-5.

Describe your physical symptoms.

What did you eat and drink?

What physically, mentally or emotionally strenuous activities did you do?

How well did you sleep, from 1-5?

Daily record   Date: _________

Rate your mood, from 1-5.

Describe your physical symptoms.

What did you eat and drink?

What physically, mentally or emotionally strenuous activities did you do?

How well did you sleep, from 1-5?

Daily record

Date: _______________

Rate your mood, from 1-5.

Describe your physical symptoms.

What did you eat and drink?

What physically, mentally or emotionally strenuous activities did you do?

How well did you sleep, from 1-5?

Daily record　　　Date: ________

Rate your mood, from 1-5.

Describe your physical symptoms.

What did you eat and drink?

What physically, mentally or emotionally strenuous activities did you do?

How well did you sleep, from 1-5?

Daily record

Date: ___________

Rate your mood, from 1-5.

Describe your physical symptoms.

What did you eat and drink?

What physically, mentally or emotionally strenuous activities did you do?

How well did you sleep, from 1-5?

Daily record   Date: ________

Rate your mood, from 1-5.

Describe your physical symptoms.

What did you eat and drink?

What physically, mentally or emotionally strenuous activities did you do?

How well did you sleep, from 1-5?

Daily record

Date: _________

Rate your mood, from 1-5.

Describe your physical symptoms.

What did you eat and drink?

What physically, mentally or emotionally strenuous activities did you do?

How well did you sleep, from 1-5?

Week 6
Celebration

Celebrating milestones and small successes releases dopamine, one of the 'happiness chemicals', in your brain. It's understandable if you don't feel like celebrating, but even in difficult times there are things to celebrate.

Perhaps a friend has a birthday or anniversary coming up? Think creatively about how you can celebrate, even if you can't be there in person. Can send a card? Print photos from a special memory? Tell then 3 reasons why you are glad to have them in your life?

What celebration is coming up?

____

How will you mark it?

____

What achievement can you be proud of? Don't compare your wins to what others can do or what you used to do. Simply think of something t is an achievement for you now. It could be preparing yourself a simple meal, showering or getting out of bed. Whatever it is, celebrate it!

What win deserves to be celebrated?

____

How will you celebrate?

____

Weekly reflections

Did you stick to your plan last week?

What was the result, will you continue?

Look back over your weekly gratitude journal. What stands out?

What new change will you try this week?

What result do you hope for?

Do you need to prepare?

Daily record

Date: _________

Rate your mood, from 1-5.

Describe your physical symptoms.

What did you eat and drink?

What physically, mentally or emotionally strenuous activities did you do?

How well did you sleep, from 1-5?

Daily record

Date: _______________

Rate your mood, from 1-5.

Describe your physical symptoms.

What did you eat and drink?

What physically, mentally or emotionally strenuous activities did you do?

How well did you sleep, from 1-5?

Daily record

Date: __________

Rate your mood, from 1-5.

Describe your physical symptoms.

What did you eat and drink?

What physically, mentally or emotionally strenuous activities did you do?

How well did you sleep, from 1-5?

Daily record   Date: _________

Rate your mood, from 1-5.

Describe your physical symptoms.

What did you eat and drink?

What physically, mentally or emotionally
strenuous activities did you do?

How well did you sleep, from 1-5?

Daily record

Date: _________

Rate your mood, from 1-5.

Describe your physical symptoms.

What did you eat and drink?

What physically, mentally or emotionally strenuous activities did you do?

How well did you sleep, from 1-5?

Daily record   Date: __________

Rate your mood, from 1-5.

Describe your physical symptoms.

What did you eat and drink?

What physically, mentally or emotionally strenuous activities did you do?

How well did you sleep, from 1-5?

Daily record   Date: _________

Rate your mood, from 1-5.

Describe your physical symptoms.

What did you eat and drink?

What physically, mentally or emotionally strenuous activities did you do?

How well did you sleep, from 1-5?

Week 7
Reaching out

It can be hard to admit when we need help and even harder to ask for it. Wonderfully, asking for help is a great way to strengthen relationships. If someone admitted their weakness to you and trusted you enough to ask you for help, would you respect them more or less?

Do you ever hide or down play your illness?

____

What are you afraid might happen if you shared how you feel?

____

____

____

What could you gain if you asked for help more often?

____

____

____

Who will you be more open with this week?

____

Weekly reflections

Did you stick to your plan last week?

____

What was the result, will you continue?

____

Look back over your weekly gratitude
journal. What stands out?

What new change will you try this week?

____

What result do you hope for?

____

____

____

Do you need to prepare?

____

____

Daily record

Date: _____________

Rate your mood, from 1-5.

Describe your physical symptoms.

What did you eat and drink?

What physically, mentally or emotionally strenuous activities did you do?

How well did you sleep, from 1-5?

Daily record   Date: _________

Rate your mood, from 1-5.

Describe your physical symptoms.

What did you eat and drink?

What physically, mentally or emotionally strenuous activities did you do?

How well did you sleep, from 1-5?

Daily record

Date: _____________

Rate your mood, from 1-5.

Describe your physical symptoms.

What did you eat and drink?

What physically, mentally or emotionally strenuous activities did you do?

How well did you sleep, from 1-5?

Daily record

Date: _________

Rate your mood, from 1-5.

Describe your physical symptoms.

What did you eat and drink?

What physically, mentally or emotionally strenuous activities did you do?

How well did you sleep, from 1-5?

Daily record   Date: _________

Rate your mood, from 1-5.

Describe your physical symptoms.

What did you eat and drink?

What physically, mentally or emotionally strenuous activities did you do?

How well did you sleep, from 1-5?

Daily record   Date: _________

Rate your mood, from 1-5.

Describe your physical symptoms.

What did you eat and drink?

What physically, mentally or emotionally strenuous activities did you do?

How well did you sleep, from 1-5?

Daily record   Date: _____________

Rate your mood, from 1-5.

Describe your physical symptoms.

What did you eat and drink?

What physically, mentally or emotionally
strenuous activities did you do?

How well did you sleep, from 1-5?

Week 8
Community

Last week you reached out and asked for support. You may have had different reactions from different people. Some of the responses may have surprised you.

This week, you will create a supportive community. Think about who has been most supportive of you during this illness. As you move forward, spend time with people who love you. These are the people who are patient and kind to you.

Who is patient and kind to you?

____

How will you ensure you see them often?

____

____

____

Who is not being loving to you?

____

What boundaries will you put around time with them?

____

____

____

Weekly reflections

Did you stick to your plan last week?

What was the result, will you continue?

Look back over your weekly gratitude journal. What stands out?

What new change will you try this week?

What result do you hope for?

Do you need to prepare?

Daily record

Date: _________

Rate your mood, from 1-5.

Describe your physical symptoms.

What did you eat and drink?

What physically, mentally or emotionally strenuous activities did you do?

How well did you sleep, from 1-5?

Daily record

Date: _________

Rate your mood, from 1-5.

Describe your physical symptoms.

What did you eat and drink?

What physically, mentally or emotionally strenuous activities did you do?

How well did you sleep, from 1-5?

Daily record

Date: ___________

Rate your mood, from 1-5.

Describe your physical symptoms.

What did you eat and drink?

What physically, mentally or emotionally strenuous activities did you do?

How well did you sleep, from 1-5?

Daily record   Date: _________

Rate your mood, from 1-5.

Describe your physical symptoms.

What did you eat and drink?

What physically, mentally or emotionally strenuous activities did you do?

How well did you sleep, from 1-5?

Daily record

Date: ___________

Rate your mood, from 1-5.

Describe your physical symptoms.

What did you eat and drink?

What physically, mentally or emotionally strenuous activities did you do?

How well did you sleep, from 1-5?

Daily record   Date: ________

Rate your mood, from 1-5.

Describe your physical symptoms.

What did you eat and drink?

What physically, mentally or emotionally strenuous activities did you do?

How well did you sleep, from 1-5?

Daily record   Date: ________

Rate your mood, from 1-5.

Describe your physical symptoms.

What did you eat and drink?

What physically, mentally or emotionally
strenuous activities did you do?

How well did you sleep, from 1-5?

Week 9
Reflection

Over the last 8 weeks you tried out lots of things to help you in your recovery. Before you close this journal for the last time, take a moment to reflect on what you have discovered and what you would like to continue in the next stages of your recovery journey.

What practises from this journal will you continue in the next stage of your life?

____

____

____

Look back at week one, are you able to do any of the things you've missed?

____

Completing this journal is a milestone, how will you celebrate it?

____

Thank you for coming on this journey with me. I wish you peace, health and happiness. Wherever you are in your recovery, I hope you are being patient and kind to yourself. Many of you will still have symptoms, you are welcome to photocopy the daily and weekly pages to continue your journey.

Weekly reflections

Did you stick to your plan last week?

____

What was the result, will you continue?

____

Look back over your weekly gratitude journal. What stands out?

What new change will you try this week?

____

What result do you hope for?

____

____

____

Do you need to prepare?

____

____

Symptom tracker

Symptom	First seen	End date

Medical appointments

Doctor	Date	Outcome

Resources

Name	Address
Perrin technique	https://youtu.be/8ESXf9PL0_Q
Loving someone with ME	https://solvecfs.org/loving-someone-with-me-cfs/

www.ingramcontent.com/pod-product-compliance
Lightning Source LLC
Chambersburg PA
CBHW031152250726
48655CB00002B/942